KIMMY TANG'S

Asian-Fusion Lenten Cuisine

Easy and Creative Recipes for a healthy joyous lent

KIMMY TANG

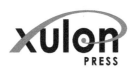

Copyright © 2016 by Kimmy Tang

Kimmy Tang's Asian-Fusion Lenten Cuisine
Easy and Creative Recipes for a healthy joyous lent
by Kimmy Tang

Printed in the United States of America.

ISBN 9781498483636

All rights reserved solely by the author. The author guarantees all contents are original and do not infringe upon the legal rights of any other person or work. No part of this book may be reproduced in any form without the permission of the author. The views expressed in this book are not necessarily those of the publisher.

Unless otherwise indicated, Scripture quotations taken from the King James Version (KJV) – *public domain.*

Scripture quotations taken from the New King James Version (NKJV). Copyright © 1982 by Thomas Nelson, Inc. Used by permission. All rights reserved.

www.xulonpress.com

Recipe Content:

Saint Euphrosynus the Cook

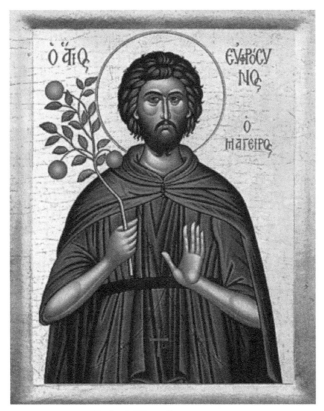

Saint Euphrosynus

Saint Euphrosynus the Cook was from one of the Palestinian monasteries, and his obedience was to work in the kitchen as a cook. Toiling away for the brethren, St. Euphrosynus did not absent himself from thought about God, but rather dwelt in prayer and fasting. He remembered always that obedience is the first duty of a monk, and, therefore, he was obedient to the elder brethren.

The patience of the saint was amazing: they often reproached him, but he made no complaint and endured every unpleasantness. Saint Euphrosynus pleased the Lord by his inner virtue, which he concealed from people, and the Lord Himself revealed to the monastic brethren the spiritual heights of their unassuming fellow-monk.

One of the priests of the monastery prayed and asked the Lord to show him the blessings prepared for the righteous in the age to come. The priest saw in a dream what Paradise is like, and he contemplated its inexplicable beauty with fear and with joy.

He also saw there a monk of his monastery, the cook Euphrosynus. Amazed at this encounter, the presbyter asked Euphrosynus how he came to be there. The saint answered that he was in Paradise through the great mercy of God. The priest again asked whether Euphrosynus would be able to give him something from the surrounding beauty. St. Euphrosynus suggested to the priest to take whatever he wished, and so the priest pointed to three luscious apples growing in the garden of Paradise. The monk picked the three apples, wrapped them in a cloth, and gave them to his companion.

When he awoke in the early morning, the priest thought the vision a dream, but suddenly he noticed next to him the cloth with the fruit of Paradise wrapped in it, and emitting a wondrous fragrance. The priest found St. Euphrosynus in church and asked him, under oath, where he was the night before. The saint answered that he was where the priest also was. Then the monk said that the Lord, in fulfilling the prayer of the priest, had shown him Paradise and had bestown the fruit of Paradise through him, "the lowly and unworthy servant of God, Euphrosynus."

The priest related everything to the monastery brethren, pointing out the spiritual loftiness of Euphrosynus in pleasing God, and he pointed to the fragrant, paradisiacal fruit. Deeply affected by what they heard, the monks went to the kitchen, in order to pay respect to Saint Euphrosynus, but they did not find him there. Fleeing human glory, the monk had left the monastery. The place where he concealed himself remained unknown, but the monks always remembered that their monastic brother, St. Euphrosynus, had come upon Paradise, and that they, in being saved through the mercy of God, would meet him there. They reverently kept and distributed pieces of the apples from Paradise for blessing and for healing.

Source from the Orthodox Church in America

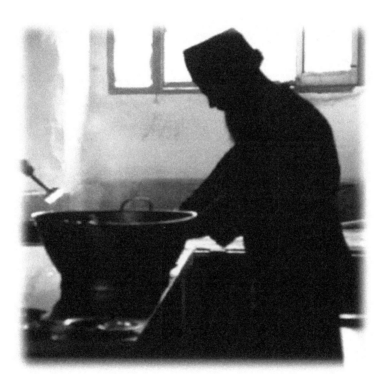

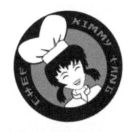

Chef Kimmy Tang's Life Story

With over three decades of culinary experience around the world, Chef Kimmy Tang is one of the greatest pioneers of Asian-fusion cuisine: combining her life experience and knowledge to create masterpiece dishes that enlighten the body, mind, and soul.

Picture a petite, adventuresome Vietnamese woman, with camouflage pants, a childlike smile, and a modern haircut. She sits on the edge of her seat, with small, worn hands clenched in front of her that have experienced years of hard work in kitchens all over the world. After a subtle sigh, she unveils her story, and we discover how a true master chef is born.

One day, Kimmy came home from school, dropped her backpack, washed her hands, and went directly to a table that she had designed at the front of their house called her "restaurant". She gathered ingredients from the family chef and started cooking under the supervision of the "safety officer", also known as the nanny! Kimmy would cook her own creative dish and invite the neighborhood children to her "restaurant". By age nine, Kimmy started to amaze her family and friends by cooking more elaborate and sophisticated meals; thus proving that she had an extraordinary and very promising culinary talent.

After a difficult time during the Vietnam War, moving from one refugee camp to another in Thailand and the Philippines, the Tang family finally made it to the United States. Kimmy lived the remainder of her childhood years in Bakersfield, California, where she continued to do what she liked most: cooking and working in the culinary world!

While continuing to grow up in America and becoming a United States citizen, Kimmy moved to Los Angeles as a young adult to further her career pursuits. Besides going to night school, she worked in a Japanese restaurant, and also enrolled at the Fashion Institute of Design & Merchandising (FIDM). In 2000, Kimmy graduated from FIDM with her fashion degree, and decided to combine her passion for the culinary arts with the elegant and artistic presentations she had developed as a fashion designer. In 2001, a brave and optimistic Kimmy opened her own "grown-up" playground, her first real restaurant called *Michelia*. Inspired by old Chinese and Vietnamese recipes, Kimmy put her own twist on many delectable recipes by introducing French cooking techniques and catering to her health conscious, Southern-Californian patrons. After running *Michelia* for 6 years, and gaining public notoriety from the press and celebrities alike, Kimmy embarked on a 2-year culinary pilgrimage throughout Europe and Asia, in search of new recipes and rare cooking techniques.

Though there have been many bends in the road of her life journey, Kimmy was baptized in the Easter Orthodox Church and came to find her true destiny and purpose in loving others, regardless of their past, and bringing joy to every person through the joy of her cooking and love in Christ.

ONION PANCAKE

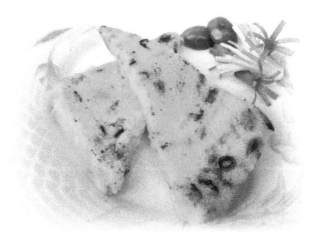

Serves 2   Preparation: 7 minutes   Cooking time: 12 minutes

Ingredients:

4 oz. green onion, chopped
4 oz. red onions
1 tablespoon olive oil
1 teaspoon cornstarch
1 cup polenta
3 cups water
1 teaspoon salt
½ teaspoon mushroom powder
½ teaspoon sugar
¼ teaspoon black pepper

Instructions:

1. In a sauté pan, add oil and onion, cook until it is fragrant. Set aside.
2. Bring the water to boil and gradually sprinkle the polenta in very slowly, whisking constantly until all the grains have been incorporated and there are no lumps. Add the cooked onion, mushroom powder, salt, sugar, and pepper. Stir evenly into polenta; transfer it onto pan. Set aside.
3. Preheat sauté pan in minimum heat with oil. Pan fry cooked polenta until golden brown. Turn to other side. Pan fry to golden brown.

"The Fast is the protection of virtue, the beginning of self-sacrifice, a wreath of abstinence... the basis of a Christian life". – **St. Isaac the Syrian**

POLENTA SPINACH CAKE

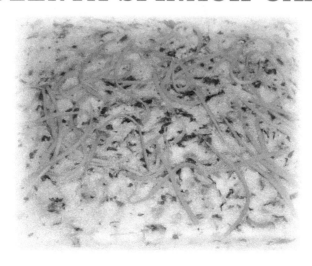

Serves 4   Preparation: 3 minutes   Cooking time: 10 minutes

Ingredients:

4 oz. green onion, chopped
4 oz. red onions
1 tablespoon olive oil
1 teaspoon cornstarch
1 cup polenta
3 cups water
1 teaspoon salt
½ teaspoon mushroom powder
½ teaspoon sugar
¼ teaspoon black pepper

Instructions:

1. Bring the water to boil and gradually sprinkle the polenta in very slowly, whisking constantly until all the grains have been incorporated, and there are no lumps. Add spinach, carrot, fried shallot, sugar, salt and pepper. Stir evenly into polenta. Transfer it to pan. Let cool, and enjoy

"Fasting is general peace of soul and body, a serene life, a consistent pattern of behavior, a way of life, pleasing God and grieving the enemy"
– St. Basil the Great

GARLIC QUINOA

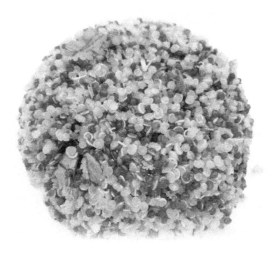

Serves 2   Preparation: 5 minutes   Cooking time: 20 minutes

Ingredients:

1 ¾ cups water
1 cup quinoa
1 teaspoon olive oil
1 teaspoon finely chopped cilantro
½ teaspoon garlic and salt
½ teaspoon black pepper

Instructions:

1. Combine water and quinoa in a medium saucepan. Bring to a boil. Cover, reduce heat, and simmer for 20 minutes, or until liquid is absorbed. Remove from heat.
2. Fluff with a fork. Stir in cilantro, garlic and salt. Serve hot or at room temperature.

"The fast is not hunger, but a little diversion from food.
It is not inevitable punishment, but voluntary abstention.
It is not slavish necessity, but free philosophy."
– St. Isaac the Syrian

KIMCHI QUINOA

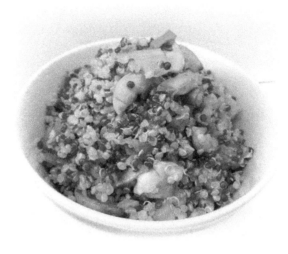

Serves 2   Preparation: 5 minutes   Cooking time: 20 minutes

Ingredients:

1 ¾ cups water
1 cup quinoa
1 teaspoon olive oil
½ cup finely chopped kimchi
½ cup finely chopped mushroom
1 teaspoon garlic and salt
½ teaspoon fresh ground
  black pepper

Instructions:

1. Combine water and quinoa in a medium saucepan. Bring to a boil. Cover, reduce heat, and simmer for 20 minutes, or until liquid is absorbed. Add mushroom and kimchi. Cook for 1 minute. Remove from heat.
2. Fluff with a fork. Stir garlic and salt. Serve hot, or at room temperature.

"Here is the Christian fast, which our God demands from us! Therefore, bring yourself to repentance, and, restrain yourself from any evil word, deed and thought. Learn every virtue, and always be fasting before God."
– St. Tikhon of Zadonsk

AVOCADO QUINOA SALAD

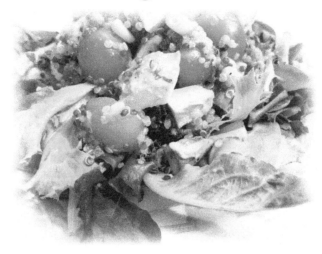

Serves 4   Preparation time: 15 minutes

Ingredients:

2 cups cooked quinoa
½ cup grape tomatoes
½ cup bell pepper, diced
½ cup cucumber, seeded and diced
1 large avocado, seeded, peeled,
   and diced
¼ can sweet corn
1 tablespoon lemon juice
1 tablespoon honey
½ cup fresh chopped cilantro
Salt and pepper to taste

Instructions:

1. In a large bowl, combine lemon juice, honey, salt and pepper. Mix well. Set aside.
2. Combine quinoa, grape tomatoes, bell pepper, cucumber, olive, avocado, corn and cilantro. Toss with lemon juice.
3. Enjoy!

"If you greedily eat and drink much, then you will be flesh; whilst if you fast and pray, then you will be spirit." – **St. John of Kronstadt**

HERBAL SALAD

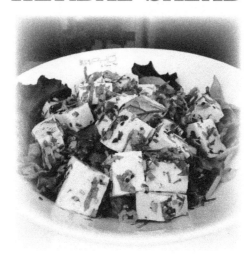

Serves 4   Preparation time: 3 minutes   Cooking time: 3 minutes

Ingredients:

1 box regular tofu cubed
½ cup chopped cilantro or parsley
½ cup chopped green onion
1 tablespoon chopped oregano
1 tablespoon fried shallot
3 tablespoons orange juice
1 tablespoon lemon juice
1 tablespoon honey
1 teaspoon sea salt
½ teaspoon black pepper

Instructions:

1. In a skillet, bring water to a boil and cook the tofu for 2 minutes, or until the tofu is hot. Set aside.
2. In a mixing bowl, combine cilantro or parsley, onion, oregano, fried shallot, orange juice, lemon juice, honey, salt and pepper. Toss it well.
3. Add cooked tofu to herbal salad, and toss well.

*"Then I proclaimed a fast there at the river of Ahava, that we might humble ourselves before our God, to seek from Him the right way for us and our little ones and all our possessions." – **Ezra 8:21 (NKJV)***

SHRIMP SALAD WITH POMEGRANATE DRESSING

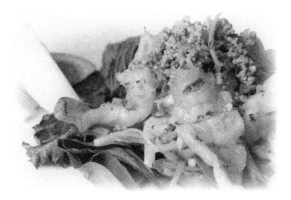

Serves 4   Preparation time: 8 minutes   Cooking time: 5 minutes

Ingredients:

1 lb. shrimp peeled and deveined
½ teaspoon sea salt
¼ teaspoon sugar
1 tablespoon lemongrass
4 oz. jicama, julienned
2 oz. carrot, julienned
2 oz. cucumber, seeded and julienned
12 piece mints leaves
4 oz. mix baby greens
2 tablespoons roasted peanuts, crushed.

Dressing:

3 tablespoons pomegranate vinegar
1 tablespoon lemon juice
3 tablespoons honey
1 clove garlic minced

Instructions:

1. Marinate shrimp with lemongrass, salt, and sugar for 10 minutes.
2. Preheat grill, place the skin side down first, grill for about 1 minute, or until it starts turning pink. Turn to other side and cook until it is done. Set aside.
3. Combine all dressing ingredients. Stir it until it is mixed well. Set aside.
4. In a large bowl, combine the jicama, carrot, cucumber, and mint. Toss with dressing.
5. Divide the mixed greens into 4 plates and then put tossed salad mix and place grilled shrimp on top. Garnish with roasted peanut.

"My heart is smitten, and withered like grass; so that I forget to eat my bread."
– Psalm 102:4 (KJV)

FRUITY SALAD

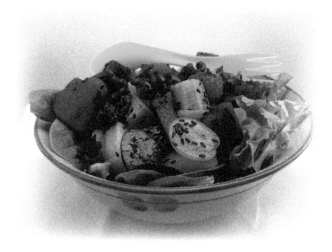

Serves 2   Preparation: 10 minutes   Cooking time: 0 minutes

Ingredients:

1 Asian pear or Fuji apple, cored and diced
5 strawberries, diced
1 cucumber, seeded and diced
½ cup pineapple, diced
4 oz. mix baby greens
½ cup roasted walnuts
½ teaspoon black sesame seed

Tamarind Dressing:

3 tablespoons tamarind sauce
2 tablespoons lemon juice
2 tablespoons honey or sugar
½ teaspoon sea salt
1 clove garlic, minced
1 small shallot, minced

Instructions:

1. Combine all the dressing ingredients. Mix well. Set aside.
2. Divide the mixed greens into 2 bowls.
3. Combine all the fruit, and toss with tamarind dressing. Place on top of the bed of mixed greens. Garnish with black sesame seeds.

"Fasting is the weapon prepared by God for us." – **St. Isaac the Syrian**

SESAME SMOKED TOFU KALE SALAD

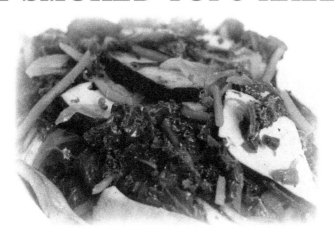

Serves 2   Preparation time: 5 minutes   Cooking time: 2 minutes

Ingredients:

1 lb. kale, washed and cut into
   1" inch long pieces
1 clove garlic, minced
1 piece smoke tofu, sliced
1 tablespoon shredded carrot
1 tablespoon finely chopped onion
½ teaspoon salt
1 teaspoon sesame oil

Instructions:

Preheat sauté pan with minimum heat. When the pan gets hot, add sesame oil and garlic. When the garlic turns light brown, add onion, and kale. Quickly stir fry for 30 seconds. Add tofu; stir fry for another 30 seconds, seasoning with salt. Can be served as a salad.

"When I went up into the mountain to receive the tablets of stone, the tablets of the covenant which the Lord made with you, then I stayed on the mountain forty days and forty nights. I neither ate bread nor drank water."
– Deuteronomy 9:9 (NKJV)

SPICY SEAFOOD SALAD

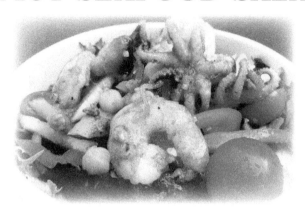

Serves 4   Preparation time: 6 minutes   Cooking time: 3 minutes

Ingredients:

4 oz. shrimp, peeled and deveined
12 oz. mixed seafood
1 teaspoon lemongrass, finely chopped
1 teaspoon ginger, finely chopped
½ teaspoon salt and pepper
1 jalapeno, diced
3 stalks celery, diced
6-8 cherry tomatoes, cut in half
4 oz. mixed baby greens
8-10 mint leaves, julienned
½ cup red onion, thinly sliced

Dressing:

2 tablespoons lemon juice
2 tablespoons sugar
1 teaspoon salt
1 clove garlic, minced
1 small shallot, minced
1 teaspoon sriracha

Instructions:

1. Combine all dressing ingredients. Mix well. Set aside.
2. Preheat a skillet with high heat; add oil, lemongrass, and ginger. Cook until fragrant. Add shrimp, mixed seafood, salt and pepper. Cook for 2 minutes, or until shrimp turns pink. Remove from heat.
3. In a mixing bowl, combine the cooked seafood, celery, jalapeno, tomato, red onion, and mint leaves. Toss salad with the dressing
4. Divide baby mixed greens into 4 plates, put tossed salad on top, and serve cool.

"Fasting is a holy classmate; fasting is the originator of all good deeds."
– St. Isaac the Syrian

SPICE CASSAVA WITH BASIL SAUCE

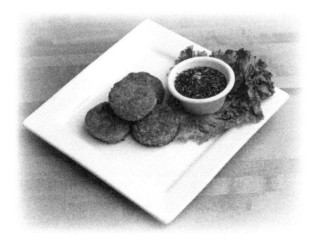

Serves 4   Preparation time: 12 minutes   Cooking time: 15 minutes

Ingredients:

1 lb. grated
  cassava (yuca)
½ teaspoon sea salt
½ tablespoon sugar
¼ teaspoon curry
¼ tablespoon
  chili power
1 teaspoon shallot,
  chopped
2 tablespoons all-pur-
  pose flour
½ cup panko
oil for deep fry

For Basil sauce:
1 cup basil leaves
1 clove garlic,
  minced
1 tablespoon
  vinegar
1 tablespoon sugar
1 teaspoon salt
1 cup oil

Instructions:

1. Put basil, garlic, sugar, salt and vinegar in blender. Blend until all ingredients are mixed well. Slowly add oil, and keep blending it until sauce becomes thick. Set aside.

2. In a large mixing bowl, combine all the ingredients (except oil and panko) together. Mix well, set aside.

3. Heat the oil to 180°C/360°F. Pinch a teaspoon of the paste, and roll it into a round shape. Coat with panko, and then drop into hot oil. Deep fry until golden brown. Serve with Basil sauce.

"I ate no pleasant food, no meat or wine came into my mouth, nor did I anoint myself at all, till three whole weeks were fulfilled." – **Daniel 10:3 (NKJV)**

TARO PATTY

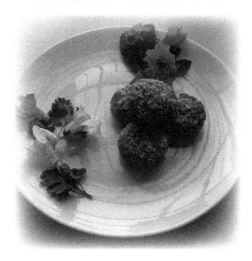

Serves 4   Preparation time: 8 minutes   Cooking time: 12 minutes

Ingredients:

1 lb. grated taro
½ teaspoon sea salt
½ tablespoon sugar
¼ teaspoon five spice powder
¼ tablespoon chili powder
1 tablespoon scallion, chopped
1 teaspoon shallot, chopped
2 tablespoons all-purpose flour
1 cup panko
oil for deep fry

Instructions:

1. In a large mixing bowl, combine all the ingredients (except oil and panko) together, mix well, set aside.
2. Heat the oil to 180°C/360°F. Pinch a teaspoon of the paste, and roll it into a ball shape, coat with panko and then drop into hot oil. Deep fry until golden brown. Serve with lettuce and herbs.

"So the people of Nineveh believed God, proclaimed a fast, and put on sackcloth, from the greatest to the least of them." – *Jonah 3:5-10 (NKJV)*

APPLE MASH POTATO

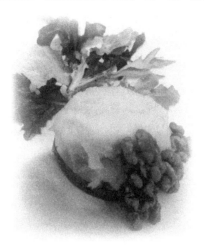

Serves 6   Preparation time: 5 minutes   Cooking time: 10 minutes

Ingredients:

1 lb. potato, peeled and cubed, boiled
1 lb Fuji apples, cored, peeled, and cubed
2 tablespoons oil
2 tablespoons sugar
1 teaspoon lemon juice
½ teaspoon salt
¼ teaspoon nutmeg
roasted walnuts (optional)

Instructions:

1. In a medium saucepan with minimum heat, add sugar and apple. Cook until fragrant. Add lemon juice and water. Cook until apples start falling part, or when the water is complete absorbed.
2. Turn the heat to low, and add boiled potatoes and cooked apples with a hand masher, slowly adding in oil. If the mash seems too dry, add some water until you get the consistency you like best. Season with salt and nutmeg.
3. Serve with roasted walnuts.

"When you will fast, then your mind will aspire and wish to converse with God."
– St. Isaac the Syrian

FRESH ROLL WITH TOFU

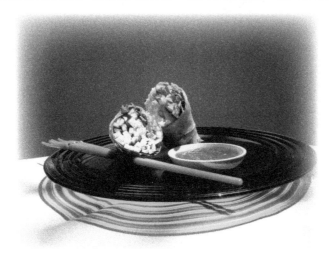

Serves 2   Preparation: 8 minutes   Cooking time: 10 minutes

Ingredients:

1 lb. grated taro
½ teaspoon sea salt
½ tablespoon sugar
¼ teaspoon five spice powder
¼ tablespoon chili powder
1 tablespoon scallion, chopped
1 teaspoon shallot, chopped
2 tablespoons all-purpose flour
1 cup panko
oil for deep fry

Sauce:
2 teaspoons soy sauce
½ teaspoon salt
2 teaspoons peanut butter
¼ cup water
2 tablespoons fresh lime juice or vinegar
1 clove garlic, minced
2 tablespoons white sugar
½ teaspoon garlic chili sauce
1 teaspoon finely chopped peanuts

Instructions:

1. Combine all sauce ingredients, except the chopped roasted peanuts. Set aside.
2. Soak rice paper in warm water. Wait until it gets soft. Place tofu, 1 piece of lettuce then jicama, cucumber, carrot and mint. Roll it very tightly. Serve cool.

*"So when they had appointed elders in every church, and prayed with fasting, they commended them to the Lord in whom they had believed." – **Acts 14:23 (NKJV)***

VEGGIE SPRING ROLL

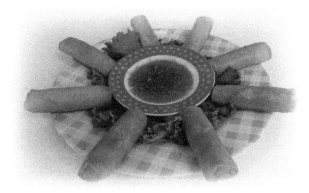

Makes about 45-50 rolls   Preparation: 20 minutes   Cooking time: 25 minutes

Ingredients:

3 cups shredded cabbage
1 teaspoon finely chopped garlic
1 teaspoon finely chopped ginger
1 cup Chinese black mushroom,
   soaked and julienned
1 cup carrot, julienned
1 bunch glass noodles, soaked
8 oz. can bamboo shoots, julienned
8 oz. can baby corn, julienned
1 bag spring roll wrappers,
   defrosted
5 tablespoons fried shallot
1 teaspoon sea salt
½ teaspoon sugar
½ teaspoon mushroom powder
1 tablespoon sesame oil
cooking oil for deep frying
2 tablespoons flour
2 tablespoons water

Instructions:

1. Heat wok with 1 teaspoon cooking oil. Add garlic, onion, and ginger. Cook until fragrant. Add cabbage, mushrooms, carrots, bamboo shoots, and baby corn. Stir fry for about 2 minutes. Add salt, sugar, mushroom powder, and sesame oil. Set aside. Combine flour with water to make paste to seal the spring roll wrap.

2. Place wrapper on a flat surface. Add 1 tablespoon veggie mixture into a corner of the wrapper, and take the edge of the wrapper, fold, and wrap tightly around the mixture. Tuck in both sides and continuing to roll up. Seal with flour mixture, and wrap tightly to the end. Cover with clean cloth to avoid skin drying out. Preheat wok with high heat. Add cooking oil. Bring to 325°F. Gently slide a few rolls into the oil, turning until golden brown. Remove the spring roll to a paper towel, and drain off the oil. Serve with green leaf lettuce and herbs.

"Fasting is a good teacher" – **St. John of Kronstadt**

VEGGIE POSTICKER

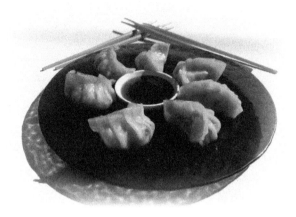

Makes about 30 pieces   Preparation: 7 minutes   Cooking time: 15 minutes

Ingredients:

1 lb. diced yuca
4 pieces finely chopped black mushroom
1 tablespoon finely chopped carrot
2 tablespoons fried sliced shallot
1 teaspoon salt
1 teaspoon mirin
1 teaspoon onion powder
1 bag of dumpling skins

Instructions:

1. Fill a pot with water. Bring to boil. Add diced yuca. Cook until tender, about 15 min. Drain it and set aside.
2. Mix all the ingredients, except the dumpling skin, with yuca.
3. Place a spoonful of the mixture into the dumpling skin, and press it to stick together.
4. Bring water to boil and cook the dumpling for 5 minutes, or until the dumpling is floating on the water surface.
5. Heat the sauté pan with oil, and place the dumplings button side down. Fry until golden brown. Serve with hot vinaigrette.

"...in weariness and toil, in sleeplessness often, in hunger and thirst, in fasting often, in cold and nakedness..." – **2 Corinthians 11:27 (NKJV)**

SAVORY SAMOSAS

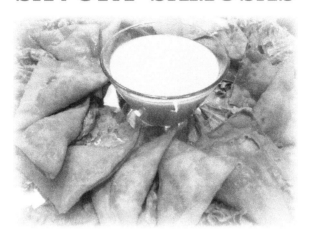

Makes about 30-40 pieces   Preparation: 10 minutes   Cooking time: 20 minutes

Ingredients:

2 lbs. yam, cooked and mashed
½ cup mushroom, chopped
½ cup onion, chopped
2 tablespoons curry powder
1 teaspoon sea salt
1 teaspoon sugar
1 teaspoon mushroom powder
1 package wonton skin
cooking oil for deep frying

Sauce:

1 tablespoon curry powder
2 tablespoons coconut powder
1 teaspoon sea salt
½ teaspoon mushroom powder
1 teaspoon sugar
½ cup water

Instructions:

1. In a small pot, add curry powder and coconut powder, salt, mushroom powder, and sugar. Slowly add in water, whisk it with minimum heat. Cook until sauce just starts to boil. Set aside.
2. Use a sauté pan with high heat. Add oil and onion. Cook until fragrant. Add mushroom. Cook for a minute. Transfer to a bowl, and combine cooked ingredients with mashed yam, curry powder, salt, sugar, and mushroom powder.
3. Place wrapper on a flat surface. Wet the edge of the wonton skin with water, and add 1 teaspoon yam mixture in the center. Press it tightly. Cover it with a clean cloth to keep it moist.
4. Preheat wok with high heat. Add cooking oil. Bring to 325°F. Gently slide a few wontons into the oil, until golden brown. Remove the spring roll to a paper towel to drain off the oil. Serve with curry sauce.

"Help me to fast joyfully and to hope joyously, for You, my Most Joyful Feast."
– St. Nikolai Velimirovich, from Prayers by the Lake

VEGAN DUMPLING

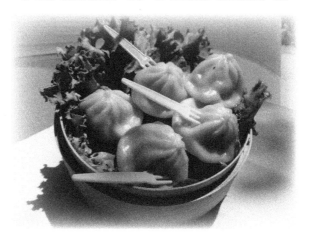

Makes about 30-40 pieces   Preparation: 10 minutes   Cooking time: 15 minutes

Ingredients:

2 lbs. yuca, cooked
and mashed
3 oz. mushroom, chopped
1 tablespoon red onion,
chopped
1 oz. carrot, chopped
1 teaspoon five spice powder
1 teaspoon sea salt
1 teaspoon sesame oil
½ teaspoon sugar
¼ teaspoon black pepper
1 package dumpling wrappers

Instructions:

1. Preheat a sauté pan with high heat. Add ½ teaspoon oil, bring it to hot. Add onion, garlic, and ginger. Cook until fragrant. Add mushroom, carrot. Cook for a minute. Remove from heat.
2. Combine the cooked ingredients with mashed yuca, five spice powder, salt, sugar, black pepper, and sesame oil.
3. Place wrapper on a flat surface, wet it with water, and fill with ½ tablespoon of filling in the center to create a pouch. Gently twist to gather the wrapper to seal the pouch and pinch off the end.
4. Bring water to boil in a steamer. Line it with a layer of cabbage or with a banana leaf. Arrange dumplings and steam for about 10 minutes. Serve with soy sauce and sriracha sauce.

"False fasting accompanies false hope, just as no fasting accompanies hoplessness" – **St. Nikolai Velimirovich, from Prayers by the Lake**

SHRIMP TOAST ROLL

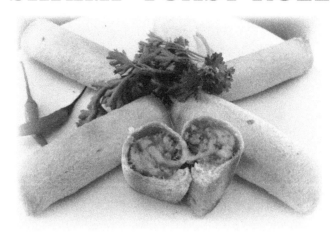

Makes 8 rolls   Preparation time: 8 minutes   Cooking time: 15 minutes

Ingredients:

6 oz. shrimp, peeled and
   deveined
8 slices of bread
1 oz. walnuts, chopped
½ teaspoon garlic,
   chopped
2 tablespoons fried shallot
1 teaspoon potato starch
½ teaspoon sea salt
½ teaspoon honey
1 tablespoon sesame oil
¼ teaspoon five
   spice powder

Instructions:

1. Preheat a saucepan with minimum heat. Add 1 teaspoon oil, garlic, and walnuts. Stir it frequently until the walnut is fragrant. Set aside.
2. Mash raw shrimp into paste. (You can use a food processer.) In a large bowl, combine shrimp paste and the rest of the ingredients, except the bread. Mix well. Set aside.
3. Lightly flatten the toast with a rolling pin. Place 1 tablespoon shrimp mixture near one side of the toast and roll up. Repeat with the remaining mixture.
4. Place the bread roll, seam-side down, on the baking tray. Bake in oven preheated at 325°F for 15 minutes, or until golden brown and crispy. Let it cool a bit. Serve warm.

"I ate no pleasant food, no meat or wine came into my mouth, nor did I anoint myself at all, till three whole weeks were fulfilled." – **Daniel 10:3 (NKJV)**

SAUTEED MUSHROOM

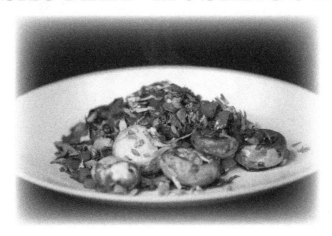

Serves 4   Preparation time: 5 minutes   Cooking time: 3 minutes

Ingredients:

1 lb. button mushrooms
1 teaspoon olive oil
2 garlic cloves, finely chopped
1 tablespoon finely chopped red bell pepper
1 tablespoon finely chopped cilantro
1 tablespoon sweet vinegar
salt and pepper to taste

Instructions:

Heat the oil in a large sauté pan. Add garlic and cook until golden brown. Add mushrooms, vinegar, salt and pepper. Sauté over high heat, stirring frequently, until the mushrooms have absorbed all the sauce. Stir in the cilantro and red bell pepper. Serve warm.

Then the word of the Lord of hosts came to me, saying, "Say to all the people of the land, and to the priests: 'When you fasted and mourned in the fifth and seventh months during those seventy years, did you really fast for Me—for Me?'"
– Zechariah 7:4-6 (NKJV)

SAUTEED SPICY SQUID

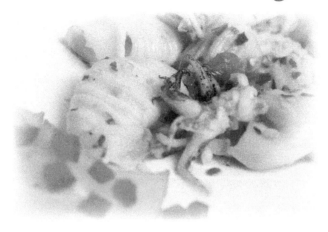

Serves 2   Preparation time: 5 minutes   Cooking time: 3 minutes

Ingredients:

8 oz. baby squid, cleaned and cut into small line, but not cut through
1 teaspoon oil
1 teaspoon garlic salt
½ teaspoon dry red pepper

Instructions:

Preheat a sauté pan with high heat. Add ½ teaspoon oil and place squid, cut side first and pan fry for about 2 minutes, or until it turns lightly brown. Add the rest of the oil and quickly stir fry. Add garlic salt and red pepper. Serve hot.

"Consecrate a fast,
Call a sacred assembly;
Gather the elders
And all the inhabitants of the land
Into the house of the Lord your God,
And cry out to the Lord.
– Joel 1:14 (NKJV)

FRUITY TOFU

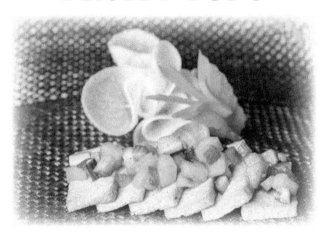

Serves 2   Preparation time: 5 minutes   Cooking time: 3 minutes

Ingredients:

2 pieces regular tofu thick sliced
½ teaspoon sea salt
½ cup pineapple, diced
½ cup strawberry, diced
½ cup cucumber, diced
¼ cup red bell pepper, diced

Sauce:

2 tablespoons lemon juice
1 tablespoon honey
½ teaspoon sea salt
1 teaspoon garlic, minced
1 teaspoon lime leaves, finely chopped

Instructions:

1. In a pot with boiling water, add salt and tofu. Cook for 3 minutes, or until tofu is hot. Transfer to plate.
2. Combine all sauce ingredients. Set aside.
3. In a mixing bowl, combine pineapple, strawberry, cucumber, and bell pepper. Toss with sauce, and put over tofu.

"Let your Lenten fasting be pleasant and pleasing to God. True fasting is the driving away of evil, the bridling of the tongue, the suppression of one's anger, the removal of carnal desire, slander, lies, and perjury. Abstaining from this is the true fast. In this fast are beautiful deeds."
– St. Basil the Great

STEAMED BELL PEPPER BOAT

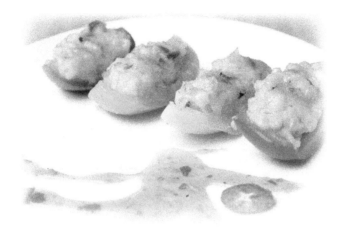

Serves 6   Preparation time: 10 minutes   Cooking time: 12 minutes

Ingredients:

3 bell peppers (best with different colors)
2 lbs. peeled and deveined shrimps
4 oz. button mushroom, chopped
1 small shallot, finely chopped
1 teaspoon salt
½ teaspoon sugar
½ teaspoon mushroom powder
½ teaspoon black pepper
5 teaspoons potato starch
optional: sweet chili sauce for dipping

Instructions:

1. Clean and core bell peppers, and cut each into 4 pieces. Set aside.
2. Pat dry shrimp and use a big Chinese cleaver to smash the shrimp, and then chop it for about 5 minutes. Add mushroom, shallot, salt, sugar, mushroom powder, black pepper, and 1 teaspoon potato starch. Combine and beat it for another 3 minutes, or until ingredients are well blended.
3. Put a pinch of the potato starch on each bell pepper, and then place Shrimp mixture on top of it. Repeat until all the bell peppers are filled.
4. Using a large steamer, bring water to boil. Place in all bell peppers, and cook with high heat. Cook for 10 minutes. Serve hot.

"However, this kind [of demon] does not go out except by prayer and fasting."
– Matthew 17:21 (NKJV)

MISO OAT PORRIDGE

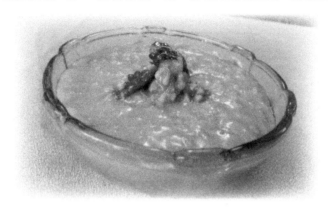

Serves 4   Preparation time: 3 minutes   Cooking time: 5 minutes

Ingredients:

1 tablespoon finely chopped carrot
1 teaspoon shallot, minced
1 ½ cups rolled oats
3 cups water
1 tablespoon miso
1 teaspoon honey
Topping: toasted walnuts

Instructions:

1. Use a mixing bowl to combine miso and honey. Mix well. Set aside.
2. Bring water to boil. Add oatmeal into it. Bring it to boil. Add carrot, and gently add mixed miso. Stir in the miso, mix well.
3. Simmer until porridge absorbs the extra water. Remove from heat. Serve with toasted walnuts.

"Thus says the Lord of hosts:
The fast of the fourth month,
The fast of the fifth,
The fast of the seventh,
And the fast of the tenth,
Shall be joy and gladness and cheerful feasts
For the house of Judah.
Therefore love truth and peace."
– Zechariah 8:19 (NKJV)

POLENTA VEGGIE SOUP

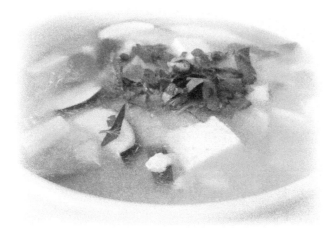

Serves 2   Preparation: 5 minutes   Cooking time: 8 minutes

Ingredients:

½ cup polenta
8 cups water or veggie broth
2 pieces tofu
4 oz. zucchini, diced
4 oz. cabbage, chopped
2 oz. carrot, chopped
2 oz. onions, chopped
4 oz. red bell pepper, chopped
1 tablespoon parsley
1 tablespoon oregano
1 teaspoon salt
½ teaspoon sugar

Instructions:

1. In a large skillet, bring water to boil. Gradually sprinkle in the polenta very slowly, whisking constantly in the same direction until all the grains have been incorporated and there are no lumps.
2. Add zucchini, cabbage, onion, tofu, bell pepper, and carrot. Bring it to boil. Add salt, mushroom powder, parsley, and oregano. Quickly stir and remove from heat. Serve hot with bread.

"The carnal fast is useful for us because it serves us in the killing of passions. But sincere fasting is irrevocably necessary, because without it, the carnal fast is simply not eating." – **St. Tikhon of Zadonsk**

VEGGIE TOFU PHO

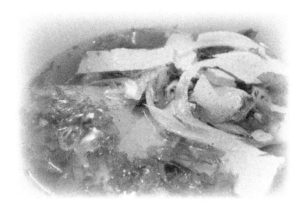

Serves 4   Preparation time: 3 minutes   Cooking time: 55 minutes

Ingredients:

1 lb. carrot, peeled
1 lb. jicama, peeled
1 lb. sweet corn
2 pieces tofu thick slice
½ cup cilantro, chopped
½ cup scallion, chopped
½ lb. shallot
4 oz. ginger (char and cut into 1 inch slices)
¼ oz. coriander
¼ oz. fennel seed
5 star anise
4 whole cloves
3-inch cinnamon stick
2 tablespoons sea salt
3 oz. rock sugar
2 gallons water

Optional: 2 lbs. rice noodle
bean sprout, basil, jalapeño and lime

Instructions:

1. Put coriander, fennel seed, star anise, cloves, and cinnamon stick into a cheesecloth bag. Set aside.
2. Put the water, carrot, and jicama in a large pot. Bring it to boil. Simmer for about 20 minutes. Add ginger and shallot. Cook for another 20 minutes.
3. Add the spice bag, salt and sugar. Cook until fragrant.
4. Remove from heat. Cover for 5 minutes. Drain the soup. Only serve broth with tofu, cilantro, and scallion
5. Best if served with rice noodle, bean sprouts, basil, lime, and jalapeno.

"Fasting hastens my preparation for Your coming, the sole expectation of my days and nights." – **St. Nikolai Velimirovich, Prayers by the Lake**

SHRIMP AND TOMATO SOUP

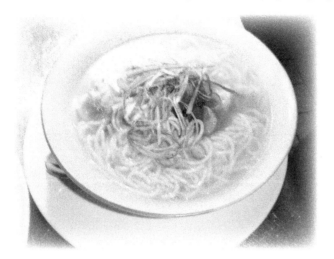

Serves 4   Preparation time: 3 minutes   Cooking time: 18 minutes

Ingredients:

1 lb. shrimp, peeled and deveined
8 cups veggie broth
1 lb. tomatoes, cut into pieces
1 teaspoon cooking oil
1 clove garlic, finely chopped
1 shallot, finely chopped
1 tablespoon crab paste
½ teaspoon salt
¼ teaspoon sugar
1 lb. cooked rice noodle
1 stalk green onion, thin sliced

Instructions:

1. Preheat a large pot with high heat. Add oil, garlic, and shallot. Cook until it becomes fragrant.
2. Add crab paste. Stir fry for 1 minute. Add tomato and veggie broth.
3. Bring broth to boil. Add shrimp, salt, and sugar. Cook until shrimp turns pink.
4. Divide the noodles into 4 bowls. Pour shrimp soup over, and garnish with green onion.

"As they ministered to the Lord and fasted, the Holy Spirit said, 'Now separate to Me Barnabas and Saul for the work to which I have called them.' Then, having fasted and prayed, and laid hands on them, they sent them away."
– Acts 13:2-3 (NKJV)

41

VEGGIE CURRY SOUP

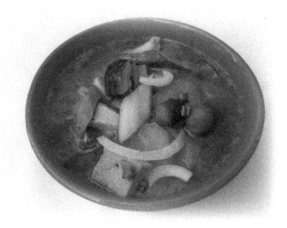

Serves 4   Preparation time: 5 minutes   Cooking time: 25 minutes

Ingredients:

1 box regular tofu, cubed
½ cup carrot, peeled and diagonally sliced
½ cup mushroom, sliced
1 cup sweet potato, cubed
½ cup zucchini, cubed
1 small onion, chopped
2 shallots, chopped
1 teaspoon chopped garlic
1 stalk lemongrass, cut into inch long pieces
3 tablespoons curry powder
1 cup coconut milk
5 cups vegetarian broth
5 cups water
½ teaspoon sea salt
3 kaffir lime leaves
2 bay leaves

Instructions:

Heat oil in a large stockpot over medium heat. Sauté onion and shallots until soft and translucent. Stir in garlic, lemongrass, and curry powder. Cook for about 2 minutes, until fragrant. Stir in sweet potatoes, sauté for 2 minutes. Add zucchini, carrots, mushrooms, and tofu. Pour in vegetable stock and water. Season with salt. Bring to a boil, and then reduce heat and simmer for 20 minutes, or until potatoes are tender, add coconut milk. Bring soup to boil again, remove from heat. Serve with noodles, rice or bread. Garnish each bowl with bean sprouts and cilantro.

"The fast is imitating angels, cohabitating with the righteous, the training for a chaste life." – **St. Basil the Great**

SPICY AND SOUR SOUP

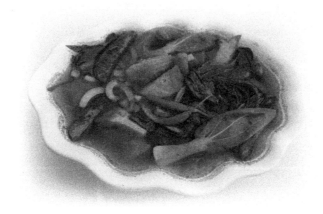

Serves 4   Preparation time: 5 minutes   Cooking time: 20 minutes

Ingredients:

4 oz. bok choy, cut into big pieces
1 cup snap peas
½ cup straw-mushroom
½ cup baby corn cut
½ teaspoon cooking oil
1 small onion, chopped
1 teaspoon lemongrass
1 teaspoon garlic
8 cups vegetarian broth
4 cups water
2 tablespoons tom-yum paste
1 teaspoon sea salt
½ teaspoon sugar (optional)

Optional:
noodles, bean sprouts, basil, lime and jalapeño

Instructions:

1. Heat a large pot with high heat. Add oil and garlic and lemongrass. Cook until fragrant.
2. Add onion and tom-yum paste. Cook for 30 seconds. Add broth and water.
3. Bring broth to boil. Add snap peas, bok choy, mushroom, and baby corn.
4. When all veggies are cooked, about 1 minute, soup can be serve with noodles, or by itself.
5. Enjoy!

"Now, therefore," says the Lord, 'Turn to Me with all your heart, with fasting, with weeping, and with mourning.'" – **Joel 2:12-18 (NKJV)**

DUMPLING SOUP

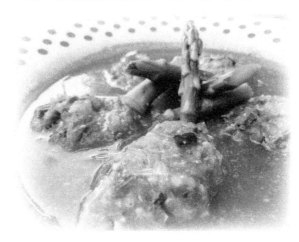

Serves 4   Preparation time: 5 minutes   Cooking time: 25 minutes

Ingredients:

½ box soft tofu
2 oz. tree ear mushroom
1 small bag of glass noodles
2 oz. mushroom, chopped
1 cup quinoa, cooked
2 oz. bell pepper, chopped
2 tablespoon rice flour
2 oz. chopped red onion
1 teaspoon salt
½ teaspoon sugar
½ cup tomato sauce
6 cup veggie broth

Instructions:

1. Preheat sauté pan with high heat. Add a few drops of oil. Add onion, mushroom, bell pepper, tree ear mushroom. Sauté for a minute, or until fragrant. Remove from heat.
2. In a large bowl, combine the cooked ingredients with tofu, quinoa, rice flour, salt, pepper, and sugar. Mix well.
3. Use a spoon, scoop mixture into oval shape.
4. Bring veggie broth to boil. Slowly add the dumplings. Add tomato sauce. Cook for 10 minutes.

*"Moreover, when you fast, do not be like the hypocrites, with a sad countenance. For they disfigure their faces that they may appear to men to be fasting. Assuredly, I say to you, they have their reward. But you, when you fast, anoint your head and wash your face, so that you do not appear to men to be fasting, but to your Father who is in the secret place; and your Father who sees in secret will reward you openly." – **Matthew 6:16-18 (NKJV)**

MUSHROOM UDON

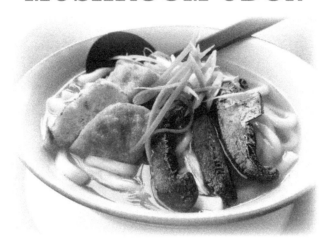

Serves 4   Preparation time: 5 minutes   Cooking time: 15 minutes

Ingredients:

12 oz. portabella mushroom, slice thick
4 bags udon
12 small pieces fried tofu
1 teaspoon garlic
1 teaspoon tea cooking oil
12 cups veggie broth
1 stalk scallion, diagonally cut
1 small carrot, julienned
¼ teaspoon sea salt

Instructions:

1. Pre heat sauté pan with high heat. Add oil and garlic. Cook until fragrant.
2. Add mushroom. Pan fry for 1 minute, or until brown. Sprinkle some sea salt, turn over to cook other side for another minute. Set aside.
3. In a large pot, bring water to boil and cook udon for 2 minutes, or until it is hot. Transfer to 4 bowls, and arrange mushrooms on top.
4. At the same time, using another pot, bring veggie broth to boil. Add tofu. Cook for 1 minute. Pour broth and tofu into noodle bowls, garnish with scallion and carrot.

"Now on the twenty-fourth day of this month the children of Israel were assembled with fasting, in sackcloth, and with dust on their heads. Then those of Israelite lineage separated themselves from all foreigners; and they stood and confessed their sins and the iniquities of their fathers."
– Nehemiah 9:1-2 (NKJV)

LEMONGRASS FRIED RICE

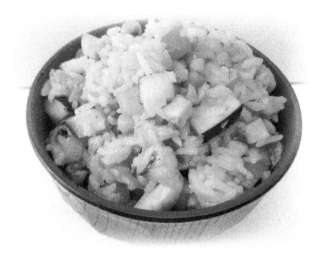

Serves 4   Preparation time: 5 minutes   Cooking time: 3 minutes

Ingredients:

4 cups cooked jasmine rice or brown rice
1 teaspoon finely chopped lemongrass
1 teaspoon finely chopped garlic
1 cup chopped mixed vegetables (example: carrots, peas, sweet corn, mushrooms)
1 teaspoon sea salt
½ teaspoon sugar (optional)
¼ teaspoon pepper

Instructions:

1. Preheat the sauté pan to a high heat. Add oil, lemongrass, and garlic. Then quickly stir-fry until it becomes fragrant.
2. Add mixed vegetables, and stir for 2 minutes. Add rice and stir-fry until all ingredients are well combined. Add salt, sugar, and pepper to taste.
3. Serve hot.

"But in all things we commend ourselves as ministers of God: in much patience, in tribulations, in needs, in distresses, in stripes, in imprisonments, in tumults, in labors, in sleeplessness, in fasting" **– 2 Corinthians 6:4-5 (NKJV)**

SHRIMP FRIED RICE

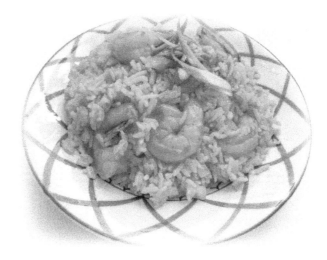

Serves 4   Preparation time: 5 minutes   Cooking time: 4 minutes

Ingredients:

4 cups cooked jasmine rice
1 lb. shrimp
1 teaspoon finely chopped garlic
½ cup finely chopped onion
1 tablespoon green onion

Sauce:

4 tablespoons tomato sauce
2 tablespoons A1 sauce
2 tablespoons soy sauce
1 teaspoon sea salt
½ teaspoon sugar (optional)
¼ teaspoon pepper

Instructions:

1. Combine all sauce ingredients together. Set aside.
2. Preheat the sauté pan to a high heat. Add oil, garlic, and onion. Then quickly stir-fry until it becomes fragrant.
3. Add shrimp and stir for 2 minutes. Add rice and stir-fry until all ingredients are well combined. Add sauce, stir fry, and make sure all ingredients are well coated. Add green onion on top.
4. Serve hot.

"Do not fast in judgment and quarrels. You do not eat meat, but you eat your brother. You abstain from wine, but you do not abstain from insults. You wait until evening to eat food, but you spend the day in judgment places." **– St. Basil the Great**

VEGGIE CURRY FRIED RICE

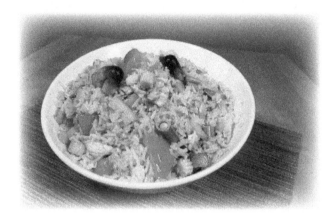

Serves 4   Preparation time: 5 minutes   Cooking time: 4 minutes

Ingredients:

4 cups cooked jasmine rice
2 cloves garlic, chopped
½ cup straw-mushroom
½ cup cut baby corn
½ cup tomato, diced
½ cup snow peas, diced
2 tablespoons curry powder
2 tablespoons coconut powder
1 teaspoon mushroom powder
1 teaspoon sea salt
½ teaspoon sugar (optional)
¼ teaspoon pepper

Instructions:

1. Preheat the sauté pan to a high heat. Add oil and garlic. Then quickly stir-fry until it becomes fragrant.
2. Add mixed vegetables, and stir for 2 minutes. Add rice and stir-fry until all ingredients are well combined. Add curry powder, coconut powder, salt, sugar, and pepper to taste.
3. Sauté until all ingredients mix well. Serve hot.

"The fast is a complement of homes, the mother of health, the tutor of the youth, an adornment of the elders, the good companion of travelers, a reliable companion of those living together" – **St. Basil the Great**

TAPENADE SUSHI

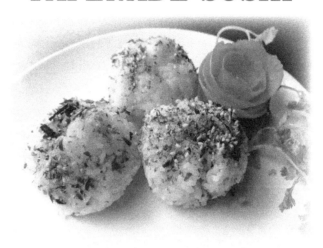

Serves 4   Preparation time: 5 minutes   Cooking time: 7 minutes

Ingredients:

4 cups cooked sushi rice
1 cup tapenade (crushed olive mix)
4 tablespoons seaweed mix
2 tablespoons rice vinegar
½ teaspoon sea salt
1 teaspoon sugar

Instructions:

1. In a large bowl, combine rice, vinegar, sugar, and salt. Mix well. Set aside.
2. Place 3 tablespoons cooked rice on a flat surface on a piece of plastic wrap. Press it into a round shape. Add a spoonful of tapenade, and tie it up like a ball. Sprinkle seaweed mix. Serve at room temperature.

"Do not, however, define the benefit that come from fasting solely in terms of abstinence from foods. For true fasting consists in estrangement from vices."
– St. Basil the Great, Homily on Fasting

IMPERIAL RICE MACARONI

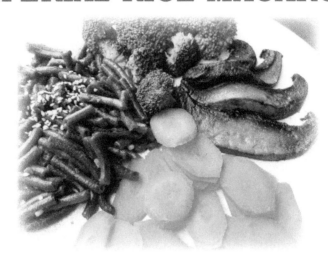

Serves 2   Preparation time: 5 minutes   Cooking time: 3 minutes

Ingredients:

2 cups cooked imperial rice macaroni
½ cup tomato sauce
3 oz. portabella mushroom, thick sliced
3 oz. steamed broccoli
2 oz. steamed slice carrot
1 teaspoon garlic
¼ teaspoon sea salt
½ teaspoon sugar
black pepper to taste
2 teaspoons cooking oil
some sesame for garnish

Instructions:

Preheat sauté pan with high heat. Add 1 teaspoon oil and ½ teaspoon garlic. Cook until fragrant. Add mushroom. Cook for a minute, or until golden brown. Turn to other side, cook for a minute. Set aside. Preheat sauté pan with high heat. Add the rest of the oil and garlic. Add macaroni. Stir fry for a minute, and then add tomato sauce, salt, sugar, and pepper. Cook for 2 minutes, or until the tomato well coats the macaroni. Serve with mushroom, broccoli, and carrot.

*"And this woman was a widow of about eighty-four years, who did not depart from the temple, but served God with fastings and prayers night and day." – **Luke 2:37 (NKJV)***

SHRIMP LO MEIN

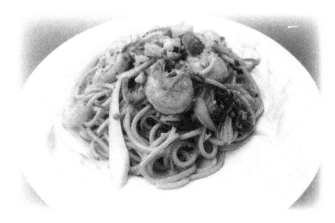

Serves 4   Preparation time: 5 minutes   Cooking time: 3 minutes

Ingredients:

1 lb. shrimp, peeled and deveined
1 cup baby clams
4 oz. bok choy, sliced
5 oz. shredded cabbage
3 oz. red onion, sliced
2 oz. shredded carrots
1 teaspoon shallots
1 teaspoon garlic
5 lime leaves, finely chopped
½ teaspoon sea salt
½ teaspoon sugar
1 tablespoon soy sauce
2 cups cooked noodles

Instructions:

1. Preheat a sauté pan at high heat. Add ½ teaspoon oil into the pan, and stir-fry shallots and garlic until golden brown, or until fragrant. Add baby clams, lime leaves, and then shrimp. Cook until shrimp turns pink. Add red onion. Cook until fragrant.
2. Add bok choy, carrots, and noodles. Quickly stir-fry until all ingredients are cooked. Add soy sauce, salt, and sugar. Stir fry until the sauce coats all the ingredients. Serve hot.

"So many are the benefits of fasting, whereas satiety is the beginning of lasciviousness." – **St. Basil the Great, Homily on Fasting**

GARDEN NOODLE

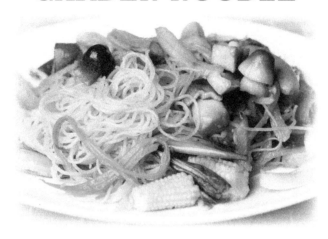

Serves 2   Preparation: 7 minutes   Cooking time: 5 minutes

Ingredients:

1 cup fried diced tofu
2 oz. straw mushroom
2 oz. baby corn
4 oz. bok choy
2 oz. carrot, julienned
2 oz. onion, sliced
3 oz. snow peas
2 oz. bean sprouts
5 oz. rice stick, soaked

Sauce:

3 tablespoons soy sauce
¼ teaspoon five spice powder
1 tablespoon agave or sugar
½ teaspoon salt
3 tablespoons water

Instructions:

1. Combine soy sauce, sugar, five spice powder, salt, and water. Mix well. Set aside.
2. In a non-stick sauté pan, heat with high heat. Add onion, and pan fry it until fragrant. Add snow peas, baby corn, bok choy, carrots, mushrooms, and bean sprouts. Cook for a minute. Add soaked rice stick. Stir it until all the ingredients are well combined.
3. Add sauce, and cook until sauce is absorbed. Serve hot.

"The meek shall eat and be satisfied: they shall praise the LORD that seek him: your heart shall live forever." – **Psalm 21:26 (KJV)**

MUSHROOM POTATO

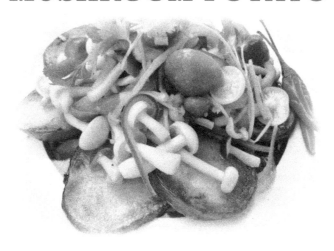

Serves 2   Preparation time: 3 minutes   Cooking time: 7 minutes

Ingredients:

8 oz. red potatoes, ¼" sliced
4 oz. mix mushroom (your choice)
2 oz. red onion, sliced
½ teaspoon lemongrass, finely chopped
¼ teaspoon sea salt
¼ teaspoon sugar
¼ teaspoon mushroom powder
1 tablespoon cooking oil

Instructions:

1. Preheat sauté pan with high heat. Add ¾ teaspoon oil, and pan fry potatoes until golden brown on both sides. Transfer to serving plate, set aside.
2. Reheat sauté pan with ¼ teaspoon oil. Add onion and lemongrass. Cook for about 30 seconds. Add mushroom. Cook for 1 minute. Add salt, sugar, and mushroom powder. Cook for another minute. Pour over cooked potatoes. Serve hot.

"Who has ever diminished his resources during a fast? Count up today what is in your house, and after a fast count it again. You will not have run short of any household goods because of the fast" – **St. Basil the Great, Homily on Fasting**

CURRY TOFU

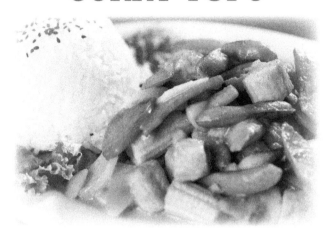

Serves 4   Preparation time: 5 minutes   Cooking time: 7 minutes

Ingredients:

1lb. sweet potato, peeled and diced
1 medium carrot, peeled and diced
4 pieces firm tofu, diced OR 1 lb. fried tofu
5 white button mushrooms, quartered
½ lb. snap peas or string beans, cut into 1
   inch long pieces
1 medium onion, diced
1 12 oz. can coconut milk
1 cup mushroom broth
2 teaspoons curry powder
1 tablespoon agave or stevia
½ teaspoon sea salt
⅓ cup chopped basil
4 teaspoons cooking oil

Option: You can add some lime juice.

Instructions:

1. Combine curry powder, salt, agave, mushroom broth, and coconut milk. Mix well. Set aside.

2. Heat the remaining 2 teaspoons oil over medium-high heat. Add sweet potato and cook, stirring occasionally until browned, 4 to 5 minutes. Add curry mix. Bring to a boil. Reduce to a simmer, and cook, covered, stirring occasionally, until the sweet potato is just tender, about 4 minutes. Add the tofu, green beans, carrot, and mushroom. Return to a simmer and cook, covered, stirring occasionally, until the green beans are tender-crisp, 2 to 4 minutes. Sprinkle with basil, and serve with brown rice.

"Fasting is beneficial not only for the life to come, but even more is it profitable for the flesh itself" – **St. Basil the Great, Homily on Fasting**

CILANTRO PRAWN

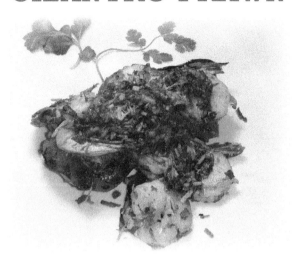

Serves 4   Preparation time: 3 minutes   Cooking time: 5 minutes

Ingredients:

1 ½ lbs. shrimp, peeled and deveined (tail on)
1 cup finely chopped cilantro
1 tablespoon garlic
1 teaspoon oil
2 tablespoons Sherry vinegar
½ teaspoon salt
1 teaspoon sugar
grilled tomato (optional)

Parsley can be used, if you do not like cilantro.

Instructions:

1. Mix Sherry vinegar, salt, and sugar together. Set aside.
2. Preheat a skillet with high heat. Add oil and garlic, cooking until it is fragrant.
3. Add shrimp. Cook for about 1.5 minutes, or until shrimp just turns pink. Add cilantro. Keep stirring it for 30 seconds, and then add sauce. Cook until liquid is completely absorbed. Best served with grilled tomato.

"As satisfying the stomach is the beginning of any evil, so fasting is the basis of any virtue and the holy way to God." – **St. Isaac the Syrian**

GARLIC EGGPLANT

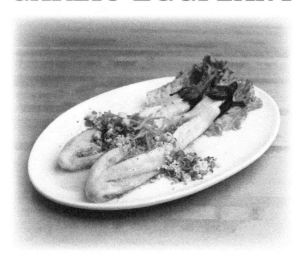

Serves 2   Preparation: 7 minutes   Cooking time: 15 minutes

Ingredients:

2 Asian eggplants
2 stalks scallion cut into ¼ inch
1 teaspoon oil
2 tablespoons fried garlic
3 tablespoons fried shallot
3 tablespoons sweet chili sauce
1 tablespoon lemon juice

Instructions:

1. Heat the oil in a sauté pan, add scallion. Quickly stir fry for 30 seconds. Set aside.
2. Wash eggplant and cut 4 line of the skin, but not too deep.
3. Using a large pot, bring water to boil and steam eggplant until it become soft, about 15 minutes (depend on the size).
4. Remove the skin and cut in half, but not through. Pour over sweet chili sauce and lemon juice.
5. Add fried garlic, shallot, and onion.

*"Fasting is the weapon for protection against demons because 'this kind does not go away, except through prayer and fasting.'" – **Mark 9:29 (KJV)***

KING MUSHROOM

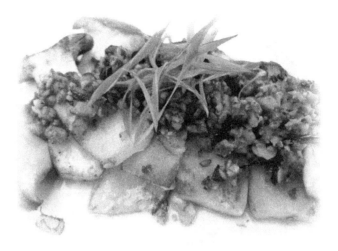

Serves 4   Preparation: 7 minutes   Cooking time: 15 minutes

Ingredients:

8 oz. king trumpet mushroom
¼ cup red onion, chopped
¼ cup walnut, chopped
¼ teaspoon garlic
1 tablespoon cooking oil
½ teaspoon salt
½ teaspoon sugar
½ teaspoon mushroom powder

Instructions:

1. Preheat saucepan with high heat. Add 1 teaspoon oil and mushroom. Cook for a minute. Add garlic, cook until the mushroom turns brown and fragrant. Turn over to cook other side for another minute.
2. Transfer mushroom to serving plate. Set aside.
3. Re-heat the saucepan. Add the rest of the oil and red onion and walnut. Stir fry for about 2 minutes, or until walnut is crispy and the onion becomes soft.
4. Pour over cooked mushroom. Serve hot.

"It is necessary for a Christian to fast, in order to clear his mind, to rouse and develop his feelings, and to stimulate his will to useful activity." – **St. John of Kronstadt**

STUFFED PEPPER WITH QUINOA

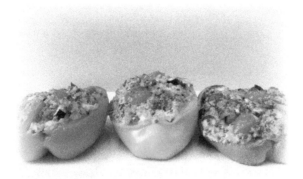

Serves 4   Preparation: 10 minutes   Cooking time: 27 minutes

Ingredients:

4 bell peppers cut in half, seeded
2 cups cooked quinoa
1 box soft tofu
2 tablespoons fried shallot
½ cup chopped mushroom
½ cup zucchini, small diced
¼ cup chopped tomatoes
1 small onion chopped
½ cup tomato sauce
1 tablespoon chopped basil
1 tablespoon parsley
1 teaspoon sea salt
¼ teaspoon black pepper
½ teaspoon honey

Instructions:

1. Preheat sauté pan with high heat, add oil and shallot. Cook until fragrant. Add mushroom, zucchini, tomatoes, and onion. Cook for 1 minute. Remove from heat. Add quinoa, tofu, basil, fried shallot, parsley tomato sauce, honey, salt and pepper. Set aside.
2. Fill the mixture into the bell pepper. Repeat it until you finish to fill all the bell peppers.
3. Preheat oven 425°F. Bake bell peppers for 25 minutes, or until the bell pepper is soft. Serve hot.

"The fast sends up a prayer before heaven, being done as if with wings, before the mountain of Ascension" – **St. Basil the Great**

TAMARIND TOFU

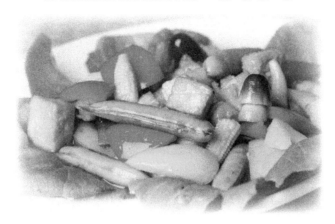

Serves 4   Preparation time: 3 minutes   Cooking time: 3 minutes

Ingredients:

1 cup fried cubed tofu
1 teaspoon cooking oil
4 oz. snap peas
½ cup baby corn
½ cup straw mushroom
1 cup color bell pepper
1 clove garlic, minced

Tamarind Sauce:

1 tablespoon soy sauce
1 tablespoon tamarind sauce
2 tablespoon lemon juice
1 tablespoon sugar
1 teaspoon garlic
½ teaspoon sea salt

Instructions:

1. Combine all sauce ingredients. Mix well. Set aside.
2. Preheat a sauteed pan with high heat. Add oil and garlic. Stir fry until it is fragrant.
3. Add snap peas. Stir fry for 30 seconds. Add mushroom, baby corn, and tofu. Quickly stir until fragrant.
4. Pour sauce in. Add bell pepper. Cook until sauce is absorbed. Serve hot.

"It is also necessary for a Christian to fast, because, with the incarnation of the Son of God, human nature became spiritualized and made godly, which is 'not meat ant drink, but righteousness, and peace, and joy in the Holy Spirit.'" **– Romans 14:17**

POTATO MUSHROOM BALL

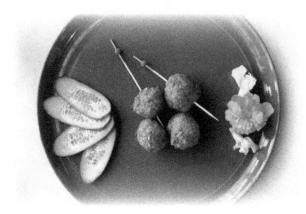

Serves 4   Preparation time: 10 minutes   Cooking time: 20 minutes

Ingredients:

5 medium russet potatoes boiled and mashed
1 small onion, finely chopped
1 clove garlic, finely chopped
1 cup mushroom, finely chopped
1 green bell pepper, finely chopped
½ cup ground walnut
1½ teaspoon ground cumin
¾ teaspoon cayenne pepper
½ teaspoon sea salt
1 teaspoon cornstarch
1 tablespoon coconut oil
½ cup all-purpose flour
2 cup panko or bread crumbs

Instructions:

1. Combine mashed potato with cornstarch, coconut oil, and flour. Mix well, and cover it with wet cloth. Set aside.
2. In a saucepan with high heat, sauté garlic and onion until fragrant. Add mushroom and peppers for a minute, or until soft. Add in the cumin, pepper, salt and stir for a minute. Remove from heat. Set aside.
3. To make the potato balls, take 2 tablespoons of potato mix into the palm of your hand. Flatten it out like a little bowl. Then scoop mushroom filling into the center. Do not overfill, because we need to wrap the filling inside the potato.
4. Now take each ball and coat it generously in breadcrumbs.
5. Once all the balls are coated, chill in the fridge for at least an hour. This will allow them to firm up and not fall apart while frying. (You can also prep them a day in advance, up to this point).
6. In a frying pan, heat oil to 325°F. Once ready, deep fry them until golden brown.
7. Drain on paper towel and enjoy!

"Reasonable fasting is a great open space for all goodness." **– St. Isaac the Syrian**

VEGGIE TOFU

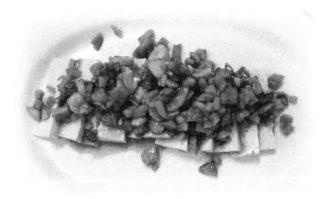

| Serves 4 | Preparation time: 5 minutes | Cooking time: 3 minutes |

Ingredients:

2 pieces regular tofu thick slice
1 clove garlic, finely chopped
½ cup mock chicken (optional)
½ cup mushroom, chopped
½ cup baby corn, chopped
½ cup bell pepper, chopped
¼ cup carrot, peeled and chopped
2 tablespoons soy sauce
1 teaspoon honey
½ teaspoon salt and pepper
2 tablespoons water

Instructions:

1. Combine soy sauce, sugar, water, salt and pepper. Mix well, set aside.
2. Preheat sauté pan with high heat. Add sesame oil and garlic. Cook until fragrant. Add mushroom, baby corn, bell pepper, carrot, and mock chicken (if you wish). Cook for 2 minutes. Add sauce and continue to cook for another minute, or until the sauce is absorbed.
3. Place tofu in a serving plate. Put cooked vegetables on top.
4. Enjoy!

"Daniel, a man greatly beloved, who ate no bread and drank no water for three weeks, when he descended into the den, taught even lions to fast."
– St. Basil the Great, Homily on Fasting

TAPENADE YUCA BALL

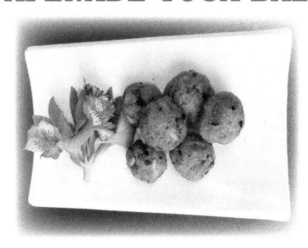

Serves 4   Preparation time: 15 minutes   Cooking time: 15 minutes

Ingredients:

1 lb. yuca, pureed
1 tablespoon cornstarch
2 tablespoons tapenade
2 tablespoons pine nut
1 tablespoon sun dried tomato
1 tablespoon fried sliced shallot
½ teaspoon salt
½ teaspoon sugar
1 teaspoon coconut oil

Instructions:

1. Mix yuca with tapenade, pine nut, tomato, salt, sugar, coconut oil, fried shallot, and cornstarch. Scoop mixture, and squeeze to ball shape.
2. Preheat oven to 325°F. Bake the potato ball 15 minutes, or until golden brown. Serve with sweet chili sauce.

*"He makes... vegetation for the service of man,
that he may bring forth food from the earth"*
– Psalm 104:14 (NKJV)

ASIAN DOLMAS

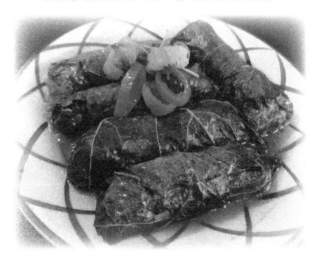

Serves 4   Preparation time: 8 minutes   Cooking time: 12 minutes

Ingredients:

1 box regular tofu
3 tablespoons fried shallot
1 bunch bean thread
  noodles, soaked
1 teaspoon tree ear
  mushroom, soaked
½ cup quinoa
1 pinch salt
20 grape vine leaves
5 cups vegetable broth
1 cup tomato sauce
2 cups water

Instructions:

1. Preheat sauté pan with high heat. Add oil and onion. Cook until fragrant. Add mushroom and bell pepper. Quickly stir for a minute. Remove from heat.
2. In a large bowl, combine tofu, shallot, quinoa, noodles, mushroom, salt and pepper. Set aside.
3. Put a tablespoon of the mixture into each grape vine leaf. Fold the outer edges over the mixture, then roll and use the chive flower to tie the roll into parcels.
4. Place all the rolls into a large pot. Pour the veggie broth, water, and tomato. Cook for 10 minutes.

"If you impose a fast on your stomach, then also impose it on evil ideas and your whims." – **St. Tikhon of Zadonsk**

SPICE SHRIMP

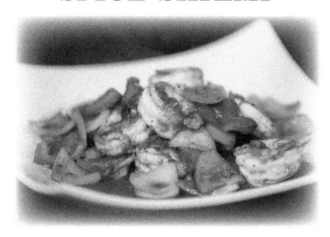

Serves 4   Preparation time: 3 minutes   Cooking time: 3 minutes

Ingredients:

1 lb. shrimp, peeled and deveined
1 teaspoon cooking oil
1 small onion, diamond cut
1 cup color bell pepper
1 clove garlic, minced
1 teaspoon crab paste

Sauce:

1 tablespoon soy sauce
1 clove garlic, minced
2 teaspoons chili paste
1 tablespoon sugar
½ teaspoon sea salt

Instructions:

1. Combine all sauce ingredients. Mix well. Set aside.
2. Preheat a saute pan with high heat. Add oil, garlic, and crab paste. Stir fry until it is fragrant.
3. Add onion and shrimp. Stir fry for a minute, or until shrimp turns pink. Pour sauce over bell pepper and cook until sauce is absorbed. Serve hot.

"The benefit of fasting is not limited to one abstaining from food, because true fasting is eliminating evil deeds" – **St. Basil the Great**

STIR-FRY SHRIMP AND VEGGIE

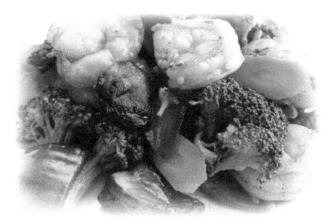

Serves 2   Preparation time: 8 minutes   Cooking time: 3 minutes

Ingredients:

8 oz. shrimp, peeled and deveined
3 oz. portabella mushroom
2 oz. red onion, diced
3 oz. broccoli
2 oz. carrot, sliced
½ teaspoon garlic

Sauce:

2 tablespoons soy sauce
½ teaspoon agave or sugar
¼ teaspoon sea salt
2 tablespoons water

Instructions:

1. Combine all sauce ingredients. Mix well. Set aside.
2. Preheat sauté pan with high heat. Add oil, garlic, and onion. Cook until fragrant. Toss in mushroom and shrimp. Cook for 1 minute, or when shrimp turns pink. Add sauce and cook for another minute, or until sauce is absorbed.
3. Serve with rice.

"Fasting, as when the iron is dipped in water, had toughened that man's body and rendered it impregnable to lions." – **St. Basil the Great,** Homily on Fasting

CHOCOLATE CAKE

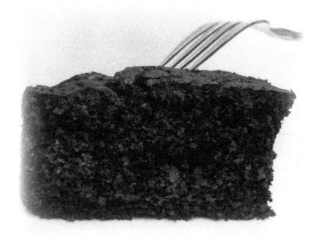

Serves 4   Preparation time: 8 minutes   Cooking time: 10 minutes

Ingredients:

1½ cups all-purpose flour
2 teaspoons baking soda
1 teaspoon vinegar
¼ teaspoon salt
3 tablespoons coco powder
5 tablespoons coconut oil
1 cup coconut milk
1 cup sugar
1 teaspoon vanilla extract

Instructions:

1. Combine all ingredients. Whisk until it becomes a smooth batter texture.
2. Pour the mixture into a cake mold.
3. Pre-heat the oven to 350°F. Bake for about 25 minutes, or until a toothpick inserted into the center comes out clean.

"And when He had fasted forty days and forty nights, afterward He was hungry."
– Matthew 4:2 (NKJV)

MANGO CAKE

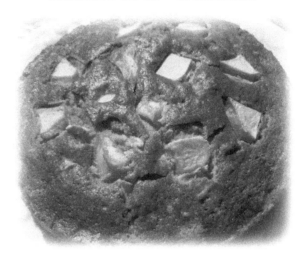

Serves 4   Preparation time: 5 minutes   Cooking time: 25 minutes

Ingredients:

1½ cups all-purpose flour
2 teaspoons baking powder
1 teaspoon vinegar
⅛ teaspoon salt
1 cup mango, pureed
½ sliced mango
4 tablespoons coconut oil
½ cup sugar
1 teaspoon vanilla extract

Instructions:

1. Combine all ingredients. Whisk until it becomes a smooth batter texture.
2. Pour the mixture into a cupcake or cake mold.
3. Pre-heat the oven to 350°F. Bake for about 25 minutes, or until a toothpick inserted into the center comes out clean.

"With fasting I gladden my hope in You, my Lord, Who are to come again."
– St. Nikolai Velimirovich, from Prayers by The Lake

WALNUT COOKIES

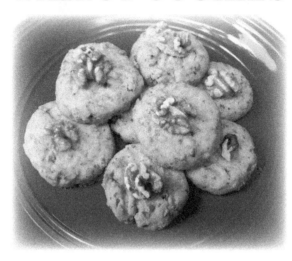

Serves 2   Preparation time: 5 minutes   Cooking time: 15 minutes

Ingredients:

1 cup all-purpose flour
½ teaspoon baking soda
⅛ teaspoon salt
1 cup roasted walnuts, chopped
6 tablespoons coconut oil
½ cup sugar
2 teaspoons vanilla extract

Instructions:

1. Combine coconut oil, vanilla, and sugar. Whisk until it becomes a smooth batter texture.
2. Add the flour, salt, and baking soda into mixture. Combine all ingredients.
3. Scoop into a small ball, and place onto parchment paper. press down into cookie.
4. Pre-heat the oven to 325°F. Bake for about 15 minutes. Let sit inside the oven until the cookies complete cool.

"So, if you will, o Christian, in order that the fast be useful to you, fast carnally, fast sincerely, and fast always." – **St. Tikhon of Zadonsk**

BANANA PEANUT BUTTER ICE CREAM

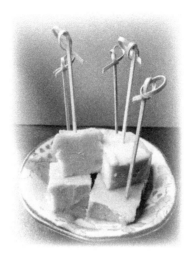

Serves 4   Preparation: 6 minutes   Cooking time: 0 minutes

Ingredients:

4 large ripe bananas
3 tablespoons peanut butter
1 cup coconut milk
½ cup sugar

Instructions:

1. Peel and cut banana into a small pieces. Combine all ingredients into a blender. Blend until all ingredients are mixed well and smooth.
2. Transfer to a freezer container. Keep in the freezer for at least 1 hour, or until firm.

"We not only should observe the measure in food, but be kept also from any other sin."
– Venerable Dorotheos

POLENTA CHOCOLATE CAKE

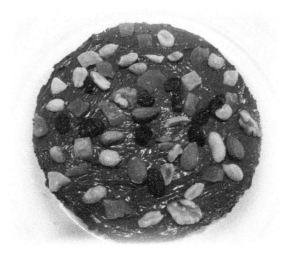

Serves 4   Preparation: 5 minutes   Cooking time: 20 minutes

Ingredients:

1 cup polenta
3 tablespoons rice flour
6 cups water
5 tablespoons cocoa powder
1 cup sugar
1 tablespoon vanilla extra
¼ cup raisins
¼ cup cranberries
½ cup dried fruit and nut mix
½ cup chocolate icing

Instructions:

1. Add water to a large skillet. Bring it to boil. Gradually sprinkle the polenta in very slowly, whisking constantly in the same direction until all the grains have been incorporated and no lumps remain.
2. Stir in the cocoa powder, vanilla, cranberries, sugar, raisins and dried fruit, and nut mix, Pour into a greased baking pan. Set aside.
3. You can serve it as is, or you can bake it for 15 minutes in an oven preheated to 375°F, or until it become golden brown.
4. Dress up with icing, and top with mix fruit and nut.

"Many fast in the body, but do not fast with the soul."
– St. Tikhon of Zadonsk

COCONUT YUCA CAKE

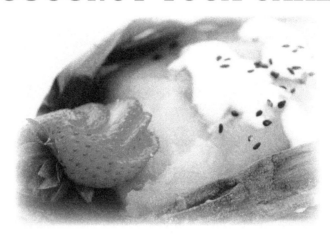

Serves 4   Preparation: 5 minutes   Cooking time: 20 minutes

Ingredients:

2 lbs. pureed yuca
2 tablespoons water
1 cup coconut cream
6 oz. sugar, or to your
   sweet taste
1 cup strawberries
1 tablespoon roasted
   sesame seed
1 tablespoon roasted chopped
   peanuts
10 pieces of banana leaf

Instructions:

1. Preheat the sauté pan with medium heat. Slightly pan-fry strawberries for a minute. Then quickly stir-fry in 2 tablespoons coconut cream. Set aside.
2. Combine yuca, water, coconut cream, and sugar. Mix well.
3. Brush a thin layer of oil on top of a banana leaf. Put about 3 tablespoons of yuca, then add strawberries and add some more Yuca on top. Fold the banana leaf like an envelope and secure with cooking thread. Repeat until all mixture is used.
4. Bring water to a boil. Steam the cakes for 20 minutes. Transfer to serving plate, then sprinkle sesame seed and peanut on top. Serve hot or warm.

"In a word: the good faster is one who departs from any kind of evil."
– St. Tikhon of Zadonsk

BANANA OAT COOKIES

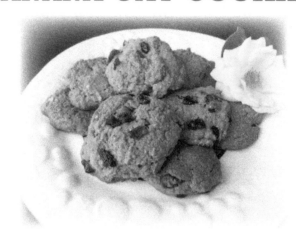

Make about 25-28 pieces   Preparation: 5 minutes   Cooking time: 12 minutes

Ingredients:

Wet:
2 large ripe bananas, mashed
2 tablespoons peanut butter
1 teaspoon vinegar
1 teaspoon vanilla extract
3 teaspoons coconut oil

Dry :
½ cup dried cranberries
¼ cup raisins
2 cups oats
1 cup sugar
1 teaspoon baking soda
¼ teaspoon sea salt

Instructions:

1. Place oats in blender, or food processor, and blend until oats become the consistency of flour. It's okay if it's not perfectly ground.
2. Combine all dry ingredients, set aside.
3. In a large bowl, combine all wet ingredients. Mix well.
4. Slowly pour into dry mix. Make sure all ingredients combine and mix well.
5. Preheat oven to 350°F
6. Form round cookies, and place on baking sheet. Bake for 9-12 minutes, or until cookies are done. Remove from the oven. Let sit until completely cooled.
7. Cookies can keep for a few days in a covered container.

"For if the Law-giver Himself fasted, is it not also necessary for those for whom the law is given to fulfill the fast?" – **St. Isaac the Syrian**

COCONUT CASHEW FLAXSEED COOKIES

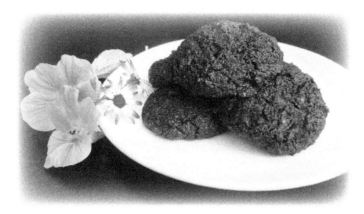

Make about 25-28 pieces   Preparation: 5 minutes   Cooking time: 12 minutes

Ingredients:

Wet:

1 cup coconut milk
1 teaspoon vinegar
1 teaspoon vanilla extract
5 teaspoon coconut oil

Dry :

½ cup cashew nut, chopped
1½ cups flaxseed powder
1 tablespoon rice flour
1 teaspoon cornstarch
1 cup sugar
½ teaspoon baking soda
1 teaspoon baking powder
¼ teaspoon sea salt

Instructions:

1. Combine all dry ingredients. Set aside.
2. In a large bowl, combine all wet ingredients. Mix well.
3. Slowly pour into dry mix. Make sure all ingredients combine and mix well.
4. Preheat oven to 350°F.
5. Make round cookies, and put onto baking sheet. Bake for 9-12 minutes, or until cookies are done. Remove from the oven. Let cookies sit until they are completely cool.
6. Cookies can keep for a few days in a cover container.

"As we fast with the stomach, we should fast also with the tongue."
– Venerable Dorotheos

FLAXSEED CUPCAKES

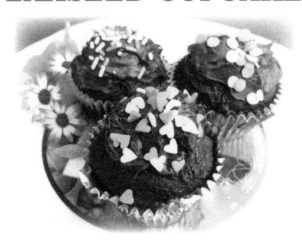

Makes about 24 pieces   Preparation: 5 minutes   Cooking time: 18 minutes

Ingredients:

Dry:
1 cup flaxseed powder
1 cup all-purpose flour
2 teaspoons baking powder
½ teaspoon baking soda
1 cup sugar
½ cup coco powder
½ cup nut and fruit mix

Wet:
1 teaspoon vinegar
1 cup coconut milk
½ cup coconut oil
1 tablespoon vanilla extract

Instructions:

1. Preheat oven to 350°F. Grease muffin and/or line with baking cups.
2. In a mixing bowl, combine all dry ingredients. Mix it completely. Set aside.
3. Combine all wet ingredients. Mix well. Slowly pour in wet ingredients to dry ingredients. Mix well, and spoon batter into the prepared muffin cup.
4. Bake for about 15 minutes or check with toothpick in the center and it should come out clean. Let it cool in pan. Arrange the cupcakes with desired frosting.

"For thou shalt eat the labour of thine hands: happy shalt thou be, and it shall be well with thee." – ***Psalm 128:2 (KJV)***

Prayers for before a Meal

Christ our God, bless us Your servants, our home, the food and drink before us, for You are the Source of all blessings, now and forever and ever. Amen.

Lord Jesus Christ, our God, You blessed the five loaves in the wilderness and fed the multitudes of men, women, and children. Bless also these, Your, gifts and increase them for the hungry people in the world. You are the One who blesses and sanctifies all things, and to You we give glory forever. Amen.

The hungry shall eat and shall be satisfied. Those who seek the Lord shall praise Him; their hearts shall live forever. Bless us, Lord, and Your gifts, which we are about to receive. You are blessed and glorified forever. Amen.

Prayers for after a Meal

We thank you, Christ our God, for providing us with Your earthly gifts. Deprive us not of Your heavenly Kingdom. Lord, as you entered among Your disciples to give them peace, enter among us, give us Your peace, and save us. Amen.

Glory to You, Lord and King! You have gladdened our hearts through Your earthly gifts. Fill us also with the gift of Your Holy Spirit, that we may abound in every good work to the glory of Your name. Amen.

We thank You Lord, Giver of all good things, for these, Your gifts, and all Your mercies, and we bless Your holy name forever. Amen.

GLOSSARY

Banana Leaf – A wide and long leaf, it is flexible for wrapping food to cook. It seals in moisture and flavor, and infuses a subtle sweet flavor and grass aroma.

Basil–There are many kinds of basil. Southeast Asian Cuisine uses the purple stem and green stem Thai Basil. Its flavor is like anise and licorice, and is slightly spicy.

Bay Leaves–Fresh or dried bay leaves refer to aromatic leaves of the laurel-like shrub. They are used in stews, sauces, braises, and soups to enhance flavor.

Black Chinese mushroom – Also known as shiitake mushroom. Before using, soak them in warm water about 30 minutes. After it become soft, discard the stems. Soaking water can be used in soups and stews.

Bean Sprouts – Mung bean sprouts are used in many Asian dishes.

Bean Thread Noodle – It is usually made from yam, potato starch, or mung bean starch. Once soaked, it become soft and translucent.

Bok-choy – A small bulb with leafy greens on top. It has a light and sweet flavor, and is often used in stir-fries, soups, dumplings, and other steamed dishes. It is high in vitamins C, A, and calcium.

Crab Paste – You can find this in Asian markets. It is imported from Thailand, and is used in soups, stir-fries, fried rice, and noodles.

Coconut Milk – This is not the juice inside the coconut, but it come from grated, aged coconut meat, which has been soaked in hot, but not boiling, water and then squeezed cheesecloth. It's widely used in Southeast Asia cuisine in appetizers, soups, stir-fries, stews, and desserts.

Kaffir Lime Leaves – They come from the wrinkled lemon tree, are a member of the citrus family. This unique leaf is a combination of lime leaf and lemongrass flavor.

Five Spice Powder – This is extensively used in Asia cuisine. It gives warm, spicy, and sweet flavor to stir-fires, roasted chicken, stews, and spice cake.

Fried Shallots – thinly sliced, crispy fried shallots are commonly used in Southeast Asian cuisine in soups, salads, or sprinkled onto to rice and noodles.

Glass Noodle – Also known as bean thread noodles, crystal noodles or cellophane noodles, are a type of transparent noodle made from mung bean starch. Glass noodles are often used in soups, spring rolls, stir fries, and salads.

Lemongrass – Produces a unique lemon flavor and citrusy aroma, and is widely used as a culinary herb in Asian Cuisine for soup, meat, seafood, and curry. It is also used as tea.

Panko – Is the Japanese variety of breadcrumbs, which is used in Japanese cuisine as a crunchy coating for fried food.

Soy Sauce – There are many different types of soy sauce form Asia, which have their unique flavor.

> Light Soy sauce 生抽 – Commonly used for cooking.

> Dark Soy sauce 老抽 – Knows as thick soy sauce. It's used for both flavor and color in sauces, noodles, and stews.

> Mushroom-flavor soy sauce 草菇老抽- This dark soy sauce with mushroom flavor is good for vegetarian dishes, if you like mushroom.

Tamarind – A tangy fruit that becomes sweeter and less sour as it ripens. It is used in sauces, desserts, stews, stir-fries, drinks, and candy.

Taro – Is a root vegetable that is often used in Southeast Asia. You can use taro as a substitute for potato. It tastes better and has better nutritional qualities than a potato. Taro cannot be eating raw.

Tofu – There are many kinds of tofu: silken tofu, soft tofu used for steaming, and mapo tofu. Regular tofu is commonly used for stir-fry and braised dishes. Extra firm tofu is good for deep frying and grilling. Spiced tofu is usually used for salads and stir-fries with vegetable.

Tree Ear Mushroom – Also known as wood ear mushroom. It usually purchased dry and must be soaked before use. Although it is not very flavorful, it adds a crisp and snappy texture to dishes.

Yuca – Also called Cassava. It has a delicate flavor, and can replace yam and potatoes. It must be cooked completely to detoxify it before it is eaten.

Dedication

Edward Aninaru – A well-known international celebrity photographer whose work includes Celine Dion, Ne-Yo, Jay Sean, and many more, accepted my challenge to …. Shoot food. Thank you for your time, effort, friendship, talent, and being my esthetic food critic. Thanks to you, the reader will appreciate and better understand a finished dish.

Reader Ray Cornelius Newman–This is a very special thank you to my friend, Cornelius, who helped me not only to crystallize the idea of this book, but also helped me tremendously to make this book become reality.

Anastasia Kalivas – A true Orthodox Christian and a great friend who was not only the engine behind the last push in accomplishing this book but also a great source of knowledge, spiritual comfort and growth.

Special thanks to all friends and family, and also to those who, in action, resources and in prayer supported this project:

- Abbott Hieromonk Dionisie of the Holy Resurrection Monastery, Temecula, California
- Abbess Victoria of the Saint Barbara Monastery, Santa Paula, California
- Father Nikon of Nea Skiti, Holy Mount Athos
- Father Eugenios of Skiti Xenofontos, Holy Mount Athos
- Rev. Fr. Calinic Berger
- Archpriest John Matusiak
- John Sanidopoulos
- Andrea Rademan
- Kimyen Tang

Bibliography

Orthodox Church in America

Mystagogy Resource Center–An International Orthodox Christian Ministry Headed by John Sanidopoulos –Fasting Resouce Page:

- On Fasting Homily I by St. Basil the Great Archbishop of Cæsarea in Cappadocia–Source: Orthodox Tradition, Volume XXIII, Number 3 (2006), pp. 6-16.
- St. Nikolai Velimirovich on Fasting–From Prayers by The Lake
- St. John of Kronstadt on Fasting – Excerpts compiled from: My Life in Christ or Moments of Spiritual Serenity and Contemplation, of Reverent Feeling, of Eamest Self – Amendment, and of Peace in God
- Fasting According with the Church Fathers – by Sergei V. Bulgakov

CPSIA information can be obtained
at www.ICGtesting.com
Printed in the USA
LVHW072234150320
650134LV00021B/2191

9 781498 483636